C000263479

Prison Health

A guide for health care practitioners in prisons

Jörg Pont MD

Rosemary Wool

QUAY
BOOKS

A division of MA Healthcare Ltd

Quay Books Division,
MA Healthcare Ltd.,
St Jude's Church, Dulwich Road, London SE24 0PB.

British Library Cataloguing-in-Publication Data
A catalogue record is available for this book

ISBN 1 85642 313 1

Note: Health care practice and knowledge are constantly changing
and developing as new research and treatments,changes in
procedures,drugs and equipment become available.
The authors and publishers have,as far as is possible,taken care
to confirm that the information complies with the latest standards
of practice and legislation.

Printed by Ashford Colour Press Ltd, Unit 600, Fareham Reach,
Fareham Rd, Gosport, Hants PO13 0FW

Prisoners are sent to prison *as* punishment and
not *for* punishment.

Alexander Paterson (1930)

Physical and mental health of prisoners is the most vital
as well as the most vulnerable aspect of life in prison.

Penal Reform International (2001)

The level of health care in prison and medication
should be at least equivalent to that in the outside
community. It is a consequence of the government's
responsibility for people deprived of their liberty and
thus fully dependent on the state authority.

Penal Reform International (2001)

Confidence of prisoners in the health care of a
prison can only be obtained if it is known to everyone
in prison that for a prison physician, nurse or healthcare
worker the patient always has to have and indeed has
priority over order, discipline or any other
interests of the prison.

Penal Reform International (2001)

Jörg Pont MD
Professor of Medicine in Vienna, Austria
For more than 20 years prison physician in
Justizanstalt Wien-Favoriten,
the Austrian prison for addicted offenders
Medical adviser to the Austrian Federal Ministry of Justice

Rosemary Wool MB BS FRCPsych
A former Director of Health Care
to the Prisons Board of England and Wales, UK
Chair of Prison Health Care Practitioners
Board Member of the International Centre for Drug Policy

Contents

Foreword

The subject of this *Guide* is of significance to every society: how to address and provide adequately for the health needs of the most profoundly marginalised members of society - those whom society excludes by deprivation of liberty. It is a recurring phenomenon in prison systems around the world that prisoners do not receive adequate health care. In many countries, the prison population is a seriously neglected group, which often is not even among the considerations of the health system. Many prisons lack even the most basic resources for health care. Yet according to accepted tenets of international law, prisoners retain all rights not lawfully taken away by the decision to place them in prison, including the same rights to health care as the general population.

The health needs of the prison population merit particular attention, not only because of the extent of the health issues presented by prisoners, but also because of the wider implications for society as a whole. As compared with the general population, the prisoner population tends to exhibit a higher concentration of health problems: prevalence of mental illness, concentration of drug misuse, higher incidence of self-harm, and a general low level of health, which makes them more vulnerable to infections such as tuberculosis and hepatitis. In this regard, the potentially negative effects on health both of incarceration itself and of the prison environment cannot be overlooked. Furthermore, from a public health perspective, it is important to recognise that most of the prison population will sooner or later be released into the community. There is therefore a public health interest in providing the proper standard of health care in prisons, particularly, but by no means exclusively, in connection with communicable diseases.

The key people for whom this *Guide* is intended – physicians who are caring for prisoners, and their nursing colleagues – face unique problems. The setting is difficult and demanding, with security considerations often taking precedence in the approach of prison management and staff. The patient population may also be difficult and demanding, from a behavioural as well as from a medical standpoint. In this context, prison doctorsand nurses face a special combination of challenges: providing high standards of health care and respecting medical ethics and human rights. Whatever the pressures and expectations of the prison systems in which they work, prison doctors are not free to abjure the Hippocratic Oath, nor can they disregard their responsibilities under international law.

It is not surprising that physicians and nurses working in custodial institutions at times feel overwhelmed by the challenges confronting them, in view of the complexity of their role and the continual development of international law and standards relating to prisons. The quality of education and training for prison doctorsand nurses varies greatly from one country to another. Even if general medical education and training is of a high technical standard in the country concerned, there may be little or no training about the special needs and challenges of working in a custodial setting, and little or no attempt to incorporate human rights and internationally recognised standards of care into the physician's training. Many doctors may be unaware of or may have no ready access to international human rights law or codes of standards (such as those established at a global level by the World Health Organization and the World Medical Association, as well as regionally, eg. by the Council of Europe). This Guide constitutes a valuable resource for tackling training deficiencies; it leads the interested practitioner from general principles through a step-by-step series of guidelines on many of the areas of work that he or she is likely to encounter when working in prisons.

This *Guide* contains many references to and echoes of human rights instruments and standards relating to prisoner health care. Although the focus is primarily on the duty to provide proper health care to all prisoners, the guidelines relate also to the physician's potential contribution to the prevention of ill-treatment by prompt and careful examination of each prisoner on admission to prison. The practice by prison doctors during the reception process should include the systematic recording of injuries sustained before admission to prison and of any account by the prisoner/patient as to how these arose, including any allegations of ill treatment inflicted by police or other law enforcement officials. Such practice may have a significant preventive effect.

On the initiative of and with the support of the Austrian Prison Department, this *Guide* has been drawn up for doctors, and other healthcare personnel, working in prisons by two doctors with many years of experience in this field. Although a single, relatively short guide such as this could not be expected to provide exhaustive detail on every aspect of prison health care, it does give practical advice on many of the problems likely to be faced by physicians caring for prisoners and it offers guidance on concrete situations often arising during their work. In this way this *Guide* can serve to improve awareness and understanding of the ethical and human rights dimensions of the prison physician's role, as well as helping to identify those areas in which more detailed and focused training may be needed for prison doctors and for all who work in healthcare teams in prisons.

Dr Silvia Casale
President, European Committee for the Prevention of Torture and Inhuman and Degrading Treatment or Punishment

Preface

Prisons exist to enforce the requirements of the courts for custodial sentences. In so doing a balance must be struck between safety and security on the one hand, and respect for human dignity on the other. An important aspect of this is the right to health care and medical services, the principles of which are set out in various United Nations and European covenants, recommendations, and declarations (see *Annex 1*). Doctors and nurses working in prisons should be familiar with these statements.

Translating these principles into the practice of health care within the prison environment can, however, present complex ethical dilemmas to prison doctors when conflicting demands are made upon them. For example, the principle of privacy and confidentiality, which is fundamental in medical care, is not, of necessity, a feature of custodial care. This short guide is an attempt to guide prison doctors through some of these situations with clear practical advice based upon medical ethics and international covenants.

The prison healthcare staff face extraordinary challenges peculiar to their work. They encounters a significantly high number of cases of drug abuse, the communicable diseases of AIDS, hepatitis B and C, and tuberculosis, and cases of psychiatric disorders, all of which are adversely affected by the overcrowded conditions in many prisons, and all of which have an important effect on the epidemiology of the community at large.

This *Guide* contains concise information on the main diseases and disorders affecting the prisoners' health.

Although it is intended for use in prison by the primary-care physician, it is hoped that it will also be of interest and of use to other members of the healthcare service team. Prison governors and custodial staff may also find it of interest to familiarise themselves with the work and complex role of the prison doctor.

For convenience the male gender is predominantly used throughout this *Guide* but it should be understood to include the female gender; no discrimination is implied or intended.

Comments that will improve further editions of this *Guide* would be welcome, and may be sent to:

joerg.pont@univie.ac.at

or to

wool1@gotadsl.co.uk

Jörg Pont and Rosemary Wool

Section 1

General Statements

1.1 The role of the prison doctor

The health and well-being of the inmates are the sole *raison d'être* of a prison doctor. The four essential principles for the practice of prison health care, as set out by the CPT (European Committee for the Prevention of Torture and Inhuman and Degrading Treatment or Punishment) of the Council of Europe are:

- free access to a doctor for every prisoner
- equivalence of care
- patient consent and confidentiality
- professional independence.

Compliance to these rules:

- promotes the confidence of the inmates
- leaves no doubt as to the doctor's medical professionalism and ethics
- prevents misunderstandings
- provides guidance in situations of conflicts
- supports quality assurance of the work
- protects against legal appeals
- gives international support.

1.2 Keep in mind

- Patients in prison have no choice of physician.
- The deprivation of liberty resulting from the conditions of imprisonment, for example loss of chosen

- social relationships and the hierarchies of prison life, inevitably increase the stress level of all of the patients.
- In prison, governors, administrators, prison officers, and prisoners may not understand the ethics of medical practice, and their requests may be incompatible with these standards. A clear explanation, suggested by reference to the documents listed in *Annex 1*, should be given for non-compliance.
- Great efforts to ensure and maintain privacy and confidentiality must be made in order to establish and maintain successful patient–physician relationships.
- Prisoners are entitled to health care equivalent to that sought after by the general public of a country. This standard must be the aim regardless of any lack of resources or overcrowding.
- Some diseases prevailing in prisoners (tuberculosis, hepatitis B and C, HIV/AIDS, psychiatric disorders, suicide) may result from imprisonment itself.
- Every effort should be made to build up and maintain a credible basis of confidence by prisoners in the prison physician and the prison healthcare service. From the first point of contact, a prison doctor or nurse should consistently make clear that the consultation process is confidential to medical personnel.
- The work of a health care practitioner is both challenging and of great sociological importance. Prisons play an important role in the public health of the community at large and are epidemiological foci for

transmissible diseases such as tuberculosis, hepatitis B and C, and HIV/AIDS. Each prison should have a strategy for the prevention, screening, diagnosis and treatment of these diseases, and plans should be in place to ensure continuity of treatment after transfer or release from prison.

- The work of a prison doctor and all prison healthcare staff is of great importance, and every effort should be made to raise its professional status.

Prison Health

Section 2

Guidelines

2.1 Primary task

It should be made plain from the very start to the patients, to the staff, and to the prison governor that the prison doctor's primary task is the medical care of the inmates and that all work is carried out on the basis of the strict medical and ethical principles of medical professionalism, independence and equivalence and confidentiality of care.

2.2 Unrestricted access to a doctor

Make sure that every inmate has unrestricted access to a doctor at all times. A patient booklet detailing the health-care services available to all prisoners (and issued to every prisoner on entry to the prison) and a letterbox for use by inmates to make appointments to see a doctor and to be opened only by healthcare staff, are useful ways of ensuring unrestricted access to the doctor.

It is the prison doctor's responsibility to arrange alternative medical cover for his absences.

2.3 Consultations

Carry out consultations on a confidential basis. If the presence of an officer is required on the grounds of safety or security, then the officer should stay out of ear-shot, and out of sight of any physical examination. Any patient contact should be documented in the medical file, with the date, the reason for the consultation, the findings, the treatment and the doctor's signature (*section 2.5*). In cases where there are language barriers, and with the consent of the patient, an interpreter should be asked for.

2.4 Reception medical examination

The reception medical examination should be carried out without undue delay. If personally unable to see each admission within 24 hours, the doctor must ensure that a nurse will do so.

The doctor or nurse must introduce himself to the new patient, giving his name and his position. The examination must pay special attention to any:

- mental disorders (*section 3.4*)
- suicidal risk factors (*section 3.6*)
- withdrawal syndromes (*section 3.1*)
- signs of violence (*section 3.3*)
- contagious diseases and high risk factors (*section 3.2*)
- chronic disorders.

All results are documented in the patient's medical file.

The reception medical examination can be used to inform the inmate of:

- the doctor's or nurse's professional independence and confidentiality
- the patient's rights and responsibilities regarding his health

- how, when, where, and from whom to get help and advice
- the risks of transmissible diseases in prison and how to avoid them (*section 3.2*).

The doctor should issue an invitation for screening examinations for tuberculosis, HIV, and hepatitis B and C (*section 3.2*).

Information brochures and audiovisual aids in several languages are helpful for propagating health promotion programmes.

2.5 Medical file documentation

A medical file should be opened and maintained for each patient. It should document a full medical history, all consultations, the prison doctor's findings and the treatment. All entries should be signed. Of particular importance is the careful and detailed documentation of:

- the examination on admission (*section 2.4*)
- information on serious diagnoses
- medical emergencies
- information on examinations and treatments with possible unwanted side-effects (*section 2.6*)
- informed consent and non-consent or refusal of a recommended examination or treatment (*section 2.6*)
- any signs of violence (*section 3.3*)
- any circumstance when medical confidentiality has of necessity been breached (*section 2.16*).

Each patient should receive explanations of diagnoses, prognoses, treatment recommendations, treatment alternatives, side-effects of treatment, and any risks of non-treatment, so that they can give informed consent or non-consent. The fact that this has been done must be documented (*section 2.6*).

In each country, every prison should have uniform medical files. Only physicians and nurses who are bound by medical confidentiality may have access to the medical files. If a patient asks to look at his file then the doctor should accede to this request. When transferred, the medical record should accompany the inmate. When released, the receiving doctor should (with the permission of the inmate) be informed of any significant information relevant to future medical treatment, and may request details from the records if he so desires. Following a prisoner's discharge, the medical records must be retained by the prison service for the time specified by the law of the country concerned. This is usually at least 10 years.

2.6 Informed consent

The prison doctor should never carry out examinations or treatments without the informed consent of the patient. This also applies to prisoners who are on hunger strike (*section 3.8*). In cases of non-consent or refusal, the doctor should make sure that the patient understands the implications of his decision, if necessary with the aid of an interpreter. Documentation should include the refusal of the patient, his capacity to understand the implications of his refusal, and the patient should be asked for a written statement of his refusal. The patient should be informed that he can revoke his decision at any time.

Consent can only be waived if this is to comply with the law, for example in the case of mentally ill patients who do not have the capacity to understand the consequences at the time, or in the case of emergency treatment of unconscious patients.

2.7 Transfer or discharges

The doctor can insist that he is told of any planned transfers or discharges well in advance, so allowing time for passing on medical information, as detailed above (*sections 2.5, 3.1, 3.2, 3.4*).

2.8 Equivalence of care

Examples of equivalence of care include free access of patients to a dental surgeon, psychiatrist, and other specialist doctors; and to the same preventive, diagnostic, therapeutic, and nursing facilities as patients in the community.

2.9 Sufficient number of physicians and nurses

A sufficient number of competent physicians and qualified nurses must be employed to care for the needs of all prisoners. Continuing professional training should be arranged, and their level of pay should not be lower than that of physicians or nurses working in other public health sectors. Professional healthcare responsibilities must not be delegated to untrained personnel, or to any prisoner.

2.10 Teamwork

Multidisciplinary teamwork of all physicians and nurses is recommended, with regular team meetings. This prevents misunderstandings and prevents mixed messages being passed on to the patient or to discipline staff.

2.11 Admission to an outside hospital

Admission of a patient to an outside hospital must be decided solely on clinical grounds. Security considerations should not be allowed to interfere with that clinical decision. In the case of high-security prisoners, when the authorities are very concerned about breaches in security it is helpful to ask a specialist to visit the prison to give a second opinion to confirm the necessity of transfer to hospital for treatment. If hospitalisation is necessary, the prison governor has the responsibility for ensuring that this happens and for taking care of security arrangements. Cooperation with neighbouring hospitals should be cultivated so that they, too, may be prepared to admit any prisoners, even those in the high-security bracket. Examinations and treatments for which prison doctors do not have either the experience or the facilities should not take place in prison. Babies should not be delivered in prison.

2.12 Prison pharmacopoeia

In consultation with a pharmaceutical adviser, the doctor should arrange for a prison pharmacopoeia to be made available to all healthcare personnel. The prescribing of medicines is the sole prerogative of the doctor, the dispensing of medicine is the responsibility of the pharmacist, and the administration is the responsibility of the nurse. All medicines should be dispensed as far as is possible to the individual patient, in a form that is appropriate to the specific patient (eg in liquid form) and should be individually labelled. The doctor will give instructions when a patient should be observed by a nurse when taking his medication. Stocks of drugs should not be held; only sufficient drugs for emergency use should be held.

2.13 Emergency kit

Each prison should have an emergency kit ready and available for the use of healthcare staff at all times.

2.14 Training of staff

The prison doctor should seek permission from the governor for all staff (healthcare and discipline) to receive training on transmissible infections, such as tuberculosis, HIV/AIDS, hepatitis B and C, on the risks of infection in prison, and on first aid, as well as on emergency management in psychiatric crises. Due attention must be given to the worries and fears of staff, and the doctor must be prepared to answer questions and offer support, and should encourage cooperation between prison officers and the healthcare services.

2.15 Nutrition, hygiene, sanitation, and environmental care

The prison doctor should arrange regular meetings with the governor to advise on all aspects of nutrition, hygiene, sanitation and environmental care (eg. smoke-free areas) in the prison. If necessary, the governor should be persuaded of the advisability of cooperating with the public health authorities. The governor should know that the prison doctor has an obligation to inform the public health authority of all notifiable diseases and any environmental concerns. The doctor must always document any advice that he gives. He should keep statistical records on all aspects of the healthcare services, including specific diseases such as tuberculosis, outbreaks of dysentery, and known cases of hepatitis and HIV, and also the numbers of drug users entering the prison (*sections 3.1, 3.2*). Such statistics help support financial budgeting, in addition to supporting the implementation and evaluation of health promotion and health prevention programmes.

2.16 Disclosure of patient-related data

Prison doctors or nurses must never sanction the disclosure of patient-related medical data to the prison administration without the explicit consent of the patient. This also applies to prisoners who have been discharged from prison custody. Exceptions to this rule include an order from a court of law, in which case the doctor should personally hand over the information directly to the judge; or an admission by a patient to a previous serious crime such as homicide or rape, in which case it is advisable to seek advice from a medical defence organisation before passing on information to the police; or deliberate failure on the part of a prisoner infected with HIV or the hepatitis viruses to inform any partners of the fact. Again if the patient cannot be persuaded to inform those he may have infected or may infect by his behaviour in the future, the doctor should consult a medical defence agency, and inform the prisoner accordingly. This is an example when medical confidentiality may have to be breached, but such a case is a rare occurrence (*sections 2.5, 3.2, 3.3*).

2.17 Segregations and restrictions

Prison doctors should not collude in moves to segregate or restrict the movement of a prisoner except on purely medical grounds.

2.18 Body searches

Prison doctors and nurses should not carry out body searches (oral, rectal, vaginal), blood, or urine tests for drug metabolites, or any other examinations except on medical grounds and with the consent of the patient. If the prisoner asks for a particular examination so that he can prove his innocence then this should be performed by a doctor who is not in a professional relationship with him.

2.19 Forensic certificates

Prison doctors should not issue forensic certificates or reports on their patients for the court or the prison administration unless ordered by the court to do so.

2.20 Disciplinary confinement or punishment

Prison doctors should not certify a prisoner fit for disciplinary confinement or punishment. And they should never be complicit in any way (even by their presence) to physical or capital punishment. However, it is important to visit every prisoner confined as soon as possible after the order has taken effect, and thereafter on a daily basis, to assess their physical and mental state and determine any deterioration in their well-being. It is also important to visit segregated prisoners on a regular basis.

2.21 Non-medical relationships

Prison doctors and nurses should not become involved in any relationships with prisoners or custodial staff that are not directly related to their professional role.

2.22 Obstruction of clinical work

If the doctor's clinical work with patients is obstructed in any way by the prison hierarchy, the fact should be documented in the patient's medical record and advice sought from a higher authority, either within the prison service or, failing that, from his professional body or an independent inspectorate.

2.23 The prison doctors and nurses associations

Support can be sought from national or international prison doctors associations. Nurses may seek support from their own prison associations where they exist.

Section 3

Common Prison Healthcare Problems

3.1 Drug misuse and dependency

Reports indicate that up to 70% of inmates in European prisons misuse illegal and legally addictive substances that affect the central nervous system, and/or are dependent on such drugs. These percentages are much higher than those seen in the general public. There is no doubt that much petty crime is committed by drug users who are dependent on drugs, to help fund their drug habit.

On admission into custody many drug-dependent prisoners are malnourished and in poor health. Up to 75% of intravenous drug users are infected with hepatitis C, and many with hepatitis B and HIV. Most new cases of HIV in eastern European countries are intravenous drug users. An increasing percentage of HIV-infected prisoners become infected with tuberculosis.

Reports reveal that:

* a majority of drug users continue to use illegal drugs in prison
* up to 79% of intravenous drug users inject during detention; in many prisons the lack of sterilising equipment increases the risk of disease transmission (hepatitis B and C and HIV may be transmitted in this way)
* up to 5% of intravenous drug users start injecting drugs while in prison.

Apart from the increased risk of infection, users of illegal drugs in prison run the risk of getting into debt, with subsequent threats of bullying, violence, and paid or coercive sex work. Threats to their relatives are also common (*section 3. 7*).

Drug strategy

In order to control drug misuse, every prison should have a drug strategy, the implementation of which is the responsibility of all prison staff. The drug strategy should include:

- measures to reduce the supply of illegal drugs
- measures to reduce the demand of illegal drugs
- treatment programmes for those dependent on drugs
- harm-reduction measures for those who use drugs, and for their associates (*section 3.2*).

Reducing the supply of drugs

This is primarily the task of the prison staff, and involves searching inmates and visitors, and often the use of sniffer dogs. Reduction in supply may also be aided by doctors in their prescribing habits. Benzodiazepines are drugs which quickly lead to dependency, and consequently are in great demand, and may be traded by those who are prescribed them. Consequently they should be prescribed with great caution and are not, for example, suitable for the treatment of drug dependency, except as a very short-term measure to detoxify a patient from alcohol. The issuing of maintenance methadone for long-term opiate users, whilst recommended, must be closely supervised by nursing staff in order to prevent methadone getting into the illegal drug chain.

Reducing the demand for drugs

Drug-free living units are a particularly useful means of reducing the demand for drugs. Prisoners who have been users but who become drug-free find it helpful to remove themselves from further temptation, as do others who are not users but who want to distance themselves from users. The term 'drug-free units' may be a misnomer because keeping any living unit free of drugs is a challenge. Doing so depends on the establishment of firm boundaries, incentive schemes, random urine tests, and ongoing therapeutic activities, particularly community meetings and counselling. Anyone found abusing the rules is immediately returned to an ordinary prison location.

Treatment programmes for those dependent on drugs

Treatment may involve:

- maintenance prescribing with methadone or buprenorphine for opiate users
- detoxification, followed by treatment programmes such as the 12-step programme that lasts for several months
- therapeutic community treatment
- individual or group psychotherapy
- acupuncture
- relaxation therapy.

It is common to combine elements of all treatments into a total treatment package.

Harm-reduction measures for opiate users

These are primarily:

- the availability of sterile needles
- the offer of hepatitis B vaccination
- the offer of confidential HIV and hepatitis testing to all new receptions into custody
- antiviral treatment of hepatitis C-infected and HIV-infected patients (also has a harm-reducing effect as it reduces the viral loads, and thus the infectivity, of its carriers)
- the availability of bleach solution
- an infection-control policy, including a procedure protocol in the case of needle stick injuries and a hygiene protocol for blood spillages.

See *Section 3.2.*

Diagnosing drug and alcohol dependency

It is important that the drug status of every prisoner entering custody is determined at the admission medical examination (*section 2.4*). The following information should be sought, so that any prisoner who is dependent may be identified, assessed, and appropriately and safely treated and managed:

- drug and alcohol usage over the previous seven days
- how each drug was used, the frequency of use, and the quantity consumed

- over what period the drug has been used, and how the use has escalated over time
- whether withdrawal symptoms are experienced if the patient does not have access to the drug.

Features of the dependency syndrome:

- Craving: a subjective experience of a compulsion to use a drug.
- Tolerance: increased use over time to achieve the same effects.
- Loss of control of usage: taking larger amounts than ever originally intended.
- Pattern of consumption of a drug is stereotyped and inflexible.
- Evidence of drug-seeking behaviour.
- Withdrawal: substance-specific symptoms, physical and psychic, if the drug is not used.

If possible, it is advisable for every prison healthcare department to have access to a specialist in addictive behaviour to help with training, and advice on prescribing. Nevertheless, it is important that prison doctors and nurses are familiar with certain basics such as identification of those who are dependent, assessment, and immediate treatment. Prison doctors need to make themselves familiar with how drugs are packaged in their own country, and the cost of illegal drugs, in order to calculate the quantities used. It is common for illegal heroin to be sold in third-of-a-gram or half-gram packages; it may be smoked, inhaled from foil, or injected. Cocaine is often sold as crack cocaine in rocks, which are heated and the vapour inhaled. Cannabis is smoked. Alcohol comes in many forms and it is important for the doctor to know the strength of particular types, eg. beer or wine or spirits.

Opiates

Daily users of heroin are likely to be dependant and to require either replacement opiate prescribing or supervised detoxification. If this is not arranged, then the patient will after 24–36 hours go into a state of withdrawal, characterised by:

> cravings for drugs, anxiety, abdominal pain, irritability, cold sweats, goose-flesh, restlessness, aching bones, diarrhoea, nausea and vomiting, tremor, runny nose and dilated pupils.

Before any detoxification is undertaken, usage must be confirmed by urine or sputum testing.

The acute phase of withdrawal lasts for a few days, but the psychological dependency and cravings for the drug may continue for many months. It is advisable, therefore, to initiate treatment programmes to help drug users. This may take the form of individual or group psychotherapy or counselling, or the 12-step programme. The prison doctor will need to liaise closely with the prison governor, and perhaps spend time educating staff, in order to establish these programmes.

Cocaine

Withdrawal from cocaine is characterised by:

lethargy, depression, apathy, social withdrawal, tremor, muscle pain inability to sleep, psychotic symptoms and ECG changes. When severe, these symptoms form a syndrome known as the 'crash'.

Treatment for the acute phase of severe withdrawal is symptomatic, such as analgesics for aching limbs, propranolol for agitation, and phenothiazine for acute psychotic symptoms. Cravings for crack in particular are severe, and consequently the drug-seeking behaviour is a major priority for the crack-dependent user. As with opiates, therapy following withdrawal is most important.

Cannabis

Very large quantities of the active ingredient of cannabis preparations are required before tolerance, and hence the dependency syndrome, develop, but this does happen and will increase in the future as the strength of cannabis on the market is increasing. Withdrawal in these circumstances is characterised by:

irritability, restlessness, decreased appetite and insomnia.

Cravings are not a problem, and as the withdrawal phase only lasts a few days no specific treatment is required. Cannabis psychosis may occur if usage is high, and this takes longer to abate, due to the long half-life of the drug.

Alcohol

The drinking of alcohol which has escalated over a period of time often results in physical complications, and patients may present with physical symptoms before the alcoholism is recognised. Therefore a careful history is important. If a patient is dependent on alcohol then sudden withdrawal on entry to custody, can lead to the most threatening of all withdrawal syndromes characterised by:

> insomnia, anxiety, sweating, tremor, nightmares, panic attacks, motor restlessness, tachypnoea, hyperthermia, hallucinations, delusions, epileptic fits and delirium.

The fully developed syndrome is life threatening and an emergency situation requiring intensive medical intervention and treatment.

Benzodiazepines

Illegal benzodiazepine usage is not unusual in those who are drug dependent. Doses far in excess of therapeutic levels are common. Sudden withdrawal from benzodiazepine use produces a syndrome similar to that of alcohol, and again can lead to a life-threatening emergency situation. Withdrawal from benzodiazepines must take place slowly, over a period of months in some cases.

Detoxification programmes

Every prison doctor should take advice from a specialist in the subject, prior to writing protocols for detoxifying those dependent on drugs or alcohol. All healthcare staff should receive training to ensure they are confident and competent to manage the process. The key to good care is careful assessment and regular monitoring of the clinical state during the detoxification process. Particularly in the case of alcohol, if the doctor is not confident that the facilities and the staff he has are capable of undertaking the task, then the patient should be admitted to a community hospital.

Healthcare staff should at the earliest opportunity (*section 2.4*) inform drug users of:

- any offer of hepatitis B, hepatitis C or HIV screening examinations with proper medical pre-test and post-test counselling
- infection routes, risks of infections, and their avoidance
- hepatitis A and hepatitis B vaccination programmes
- treatment offered in the prison.

Community contacts

Drug and alcohol dependency may lead to a non-structured, non-conforming lifestyle with loss of health and also loss of social supports including work, family, and home. Many never access treatment services. Prison presents them with an opportunity to address their health problems, and to re-establish some structure into their lives, albeit an imposed structure, and to offer treatment.

Where possible, prison healthcare staff should establish contacts with community drug agencies and make arrangements for all those receiving treatment in prison to link with their community agency, so that help is available as soon as the patients get out of prison. Unfortunately in some countries there is a dearth of treatment facilities in the community, so this is not possible. It is the responsibility of the prison authorities to keep statistical information, and so prove the importance, in the interests of public health, of developing community services.

Pregnant women

Pregnant women who are drug dependent should be under the care of specialist community services throughout their pregnancy and immediately post-partum. Those using opiates should be prescribed substitute opiates which should be maintained at a similar level to the illegal drug during the first trimester. Detoxification may then be considered if that is what the mother desires. If this is not achieved by the end of the second trimester, then the substitute drug should remain steady until after delivery. Babies born to drug-dependent mothers are usually affected by the drug and develop a withdrawal syndrome. They require specialist paediatric care in a hospital unit.

Prior to release all prisoners should be warned of the dangers of returning to drug use at a level they were at prior to imprisonment. Returning to previous levels of usage could lead to a potentially fatal overdose.

3.2 Transmissible infections: tuberculosis, HIV/AIDS, hepatitis B and hepatitis C

Prisons are epidemiological foci for these infections and diseases due to the fact that:

- disproportionately high numbers of inmates come from socioeconomically disadvantaged groups with high prevalence and incidence rates for these infections, secondary to poverty, malnutrition, poor hygiene and high-risk behaviour. As these infections and infectious diseases may be undiagnosed in the community, a significant percentage of those entering prison may be unknowingly infected
- in prison, the risk of transmission of these infections is increased by overcrowding, poor hygiene facilities, continuation of high-risk behaviour, and non-availability of harm reducing measures
- constant movement of infected people into prisons and then out again into civil society explains the epidemiological significance of prisons for society as a whole.

Tuberculosis

In addition to poverty and malnutrition, the HIV pandemic is the main cause for the five-fold increase in worldwide tuberculosis incidence in the last 15 years. HIV and tuberculosis form a lethal combination, each speeding the other's progress. Homelessness, malnutrition, and intravenous drug usage increase the risk for one or both infections. Within the prison environment, overcrowding, lack of ventilation and sunlight, and the continuation of high-risk behaviours for HIV infection, lead to prisons being particularly high-risk environments for the co-infection of tuberculosis and HIV.

The increase of resistant and multidrug-resistant tuberculosis infection, ie. resistant to at least isoniazid and rifampicin, the two most effective anti-tuberculosis drugs, has greatly increased the morbidity and threat of transmission of tuberculosis. Drug-resistant tuberculosis is caused by inconsistent or partial treatment, when patients do not take their medicines regularly for the required period either because they start to feel better, or because doctors prescribe the wrong treatment regimens, or because the drug supply is unreliable. Drug-resistant tuberculosis is generally treatable, but it requires extensive chemotherapy for up to 2 years, which is prohibitively expensive and may be toxic to the patient. In the epidemics affecting prisons of Eastern Europe and central Asia, the prevalence of tuberculosis in prisoners was of the order of 20% and of this 20% around 25% were infected with multiresistant strains.

The decisive principles for the control of tuberculosis are:

* early identification of infectious patients by clinical assessment of symptoms ie. coughing for more than 3 weeks, and positive sputum smear screening for tuberculosis should now become a routine part of the reception medical procedure
* separation of the patient until a negative smear is obtained

- treatment by means of the DOTS (directly observed treatment, short-course), which includes a supervised treatment period of six to eight months with direct observation of ingestion of medication, and the establishment of a well-defined reporting system to monitor treatment, patient progress, and programme performance.

For procedural, diagnostic, and therapeutic details we refer to the *WHO Guidelines for the Control of Tuberculosis in Prisons* (Maher *et al*, 1998).

Prisoners

Anti-tuberculosis medication is in demand on the black market, and poverty may lead some ill prisoners to sell their medication in exchange for currency. Alternatively some prisoners may fake a positive sputum test by using the sputum of a fellow prisoner who is positive, in order to obtain medication to sell on the black market. It is therefore very important that the production of the sputum sample, in addition to the ingestion of medicine, is closely observed. Frequent contact between the prison doctor or nurse and the patient remains an important element of treatment in order for the patient to fully understand the side-effects of the treatment, to be encouraged by the progress being made, and to understand the consequences of not complying with the regimen (*section 2.6*).

Prison staff

The prison staff are sharing this high-risk environment with the prisoners. They should receive education and training about tuberculosis (*section 2.14*). Any member of staff who is in direct contact with an infectious tuberculosis patient should be offered the use of a high-efficiency particulate air mask. Those who are actively infected should be asked to wear surgical masks when in contact with staff or relatives.

Community links

There should be close collaboration with the national health authority and community tuberculosis treatment institution. The medication for tuberculosis patients should be provided by the national authorities, each case should be incorporated onto the national register, and treatment should be monitored and controlled by the specialist agencies both during the time of imprisonment and after discharge. It is most important that arrangements are made for follow-up in the community well ahead of the discharge of the patient from prison (*section 2.7*).

HIV/AIDS, hepatitis B and hepatitis C

The estimated prevalence of HIV, hepatitis B and hepatitis C in prisoners varies considerably between different European countries, depending upon the prevalence of injecting drug users in the country, and upon the national laws and sentencing practices for drug-related drug users and dependents. HIV prevalence ranges between

0.03% and 10%. Currently it is higher in western than eastern European states, but it is increasing rapidly in the latter. The prevalence of hepatitis B and C infections is much higher than HIV due to their higher infectivity.

In prison there is a high risk of infection by parenterally transmissible viruses due to overcrowding and the high-risk behaviour of inmates, and to non-availability of harm-reducing measures. Imprisonment has been shown to increase the risk of HIV and hepatitis C infections in drug users, and epidemic outbreaks of HIV infections in prisons have been reported. Co-infections of HIV with hepatitis B and C in injecting drug users are common, and are likely to complicate the prognosis and treatment of each disease.

Transmission in prison

Transmission in prisons occurs by:

- intravenous drug use with shared equipment
- tattooing with shared needles and ink
- unprotected penetrative sex.

Prevention methods

Health information may be disseminated by means of:

- brief intervention by the doctor and nurses at the reception medical interview and whenever opportunities present
- leaflets written at a level that caters for poorly educated prisoners

- videos as a part of health education classes and also during leisure activities
- inmate and staff workshops facilitated by community services (either NGO- or government-funded)
- strict adherence to a procedure protocol in the case of needlestick injuries (post-exposure prophylactic antiretroviral treatment) and hygiene protocol for blood spillages.

Supply can be reduced by the discipline officers using:

- regular and random searching
- random urine testing (this is controversial as there is an increased risk of the prisoner population switching from cannabis to opiates which have a shorter half-life)
- sniffer dogs.

Harm-reduction can be achieved by:

- making condoms readily available
- providing disinfectant for cleaning syringes and for blood spillages
- establishing needle exchange programmes, as now practiced safely in some prisons in Switzerland, Germany, Spain and Moldova
- offering hepatitis B vaccination to all injecting drug users and to all staff
- offering confidential HIV and hepatitis testing to all new receptions into custody (segregation of positive patients is not necessary; *section 2.17*)

- offering opiate substitution programmes
- offering detoxification treatment to those who are willing to commit to abstinence
- provision of drug-free living units
- making every effort to stamp out sexual violence that comes to the notice of any member of staff, including the medical staff (*section 3.3*); medical staff can make the governor aware of their concerns without breaking individual confidentiality.

Antiretroviral treatment of patients infected with hepatitis C and HIV also has a preventive effect, because it reduces the viral loads and thus the infectivity of its carriers.

Caring for HIV-positive and hepatitis-positive patients

It is advisable that all patients who are positive for HIV or hepatitis B or C are under the care of specialist services in the community. Prison doctors will be involved with their treatment and management because it is they who have the day-to-day and ultimate responsibility.

- Doctors are involved in counselling their patients in one way or another at all consultations. If a patient is known to be indulging in high-risk behaviour, then the doctor has a duty to inform him of the risk involved, and how these risks may be reduced. However, prior to a patient agreeing to testing, it is advisable to seek the services of a counsellor who is trained in the subject, who may be a member of the community specialist team. This ensures that the patient is giving truly informed consent to the test. Similarly, after the test counselling is required, whatever the result, to help manage the way forward and to minimise all possible harm to the patient and also to others.

■ If indicated, treatment with interferon plus ribavirin for chronic hepatitis C should be given, and the HAART programme (highly active antiretroviral treatment) for advanced cases of HIV infection should be followed. Again, the patient should be under the supervision of a specialist, and the principal of equivalence of care must apply (*section 2.8*).

■ In the case of a terminally ill AIDS patient, consent should be sought for his release, either to an institution or to his home. There are several ways in which the authorities may effect such a release. However, if the authorities are reluctant to do this, because they think the patient still presents a danger, then a normal hospital admission on medical grounds may have to be sought as death approaches (*section 3.9*).

■ Pregnant women who are HIV-positive or have active hepatitis B or C must be under the care of a specialist microbiologist (or other specialist who is managing HIV patients), consulting together with an obstetrician and a paediatrician in addition to the prison doctor. Everything must be done to reduce to a minimum the risk of vertical transmission of the virus to the fetus.

▨ It is important that prisoners are not excluded from clinical trials which are expected to produce a direct and significant benefit to their health, as is the case in some of the trials of new antiretroviral drugs or their combinations. However, their participation does raise ethical issues because prisoners generally should not be asked to participate in medical research. Great care is needed to ensure informed consent, and there should also be approval from an independent ethical committee who are made aware that prisoners wish to participate (*section 3.10*).

3.3 Violence

Violence in a prison is dependent on many interacting factors, and if it is allowed to escalate the prison may become a very unsafe place in which to live and work for both inmates and staff. Identifying the causes of violence, and maintaining the control of a prison are therefore a crucial part of the prison governor's job.

Environmental causes of violence include:

▨ prisoner overcrowding
▨ staff shortages and poor deployment of staff
▨ lack of work and occupational activities for the prisoners
▨ failure to manage ethnic, religious and even regional differences and mixes
▨ failure to adhere to a clear policy to eliminate ethnic discrimination by staff as well as inmates.

A percentage of prisoners are charged with, or are serving sentences for, violent offences. They are people who, if not prone to violent behaviour, have certainly indulged in it at the time of their offence. Many have antisocial or aggressive personality disorders, and manage interpersonal disputes or personal frustrations by violent means. They also are sensitive to invasion of their personal body space (*section 3.4*). Drug misuse and particularly cocaine misuse and alcohol can increase violent behaviour.

Prison doctors have a duty to examine and document all physical signs of violence, and to note any revealed evidence of psychological violence such as bullying, and the possibility of sexual violence. At the reception medical examination a prisoner may report police violence and it is important to reveal any evidence of this to the authorities. If the prisoner is reluctant to give permission for this, the doctor must seek ways of ensuring that the victim's identity is not revealed to the offender.

If the prison doctor believes that a patient is intent on perpetrating a violent crime against another, then the doctor has a duty to prioritise the welfare of the other person ahead of the duty of confidentiality to his patient (*section 2.16*).

The doctor should not become involved in the prosecution and punishment of offenders, beyond that of supplying factual medical evidence to the governor at the request of the offender. However it is the duty of the doctor to visit the punishment cells, and if a prisoner is receiving punishment for violence, it is worthwhile exploring with him the triggers that lead him to behave in this way. If it is perpetual behaviour, and if the prisoner expresses regrets, then the doctor might explore the possibility of offering psychiatric or psychological help (*section 3.4*). Regrettably, most prisons do not have such resources available.

The prison doctor should record all findings of violence in order to provide systematic statistics about violence in the prison to the prison governor and the prison authorities. Systematic statistics on violence can help an assessment of the situation, and can also help to evaluate preventive measures. Indeed, to do so may even have a preventive effect in and of itself.

3.4 Mental disorders

Prevalence

A review of serious mental disorders among prisoners in Western countries (Fazel and Danish, 2002) found that one in seven have a psychotic illness or major depression; and one in two of all men prisoners and one in five of women prisoners have an antisocial personality disorder. These rates are up to ten times the rates found in comparable community samples. There has been very little research into non-Western prison populations. Out of a total of some 9 million people imprisoned worldwide, only around 30% are in Western countries, whereas 99% of the available data from prison surveys are derived from Western countries.

Fazel and Danesh reviewed sixty-two surveys dating from January 1966 to January 2001, which used either clinical examinations or diagnostic instruments. Questionnaire surveys were discounted. The countries from which the surveys were taken were Australia, Canada, Denmark, Finland, Ireland, the Netherlands, New Zealand, Norway, Spain, Sweden, the UK and the USA. The number of prisoners included in those surveys was 22 790, of whom 81% were men.

Their findings confirmed that the burden of mental disorder among prisoners is heavy: 3.7% of men and 4.0% of women had psychotic illness; 10.0% of men and 12.0% of women had major depression; and 65% of men and 42% of women had a personality disorder, including 47.0% and 21.0% respectively with an antisocial personality disorder.

In addition to the major mental disorders mentioned, neuroses and drug and alcohol dependency also have a high prevalence rate in prison populations, and comorbidity is a complicating factor.

Diagnosing mental disorders

The United Nations Standard Minimum Rules for the Treatment of Prisoners, and the European Prison Rules include the requirement that prisons should have a mental health service for prisoners, which is linked closely with the community services. Notwithstanding this, it is important that the prison physician has a good working knowledge of mental health assessment, to enable him to identify those with a mental disorder, institute any appropriate treatment, and/or refer to the psychiatric team.

Assessment

Assessment must begin at the point of reception into prison (*section 2.4*). It is important that certain questions are asked in order to alert the healthcare professional, whether a doctor or nurse, who is undertaking the assessment of any prisoner to the necessity for urgent follow-up treatment and management.

Identifying mental health problems

Assessment questions to identify the possibility of a mental health problem:

- Has the prisoner ever received psychiatric treatment?
- Is the prisoner currently taking medication?
- Is there a history of suicide attempts?
- Is the prisoner currently experiencing suicidal ideation?
- Is the prisoner dependent on alcohol?
- Is the prisoner dependent on any drugs?
- Is the offence one of homicide or a sexual offence?
- Is there any family history of mental illness?

Identifying suicidal ideation

Suicide rates among prisoners are invariably high. However, given appropriate identification and patient care, suicides can be prevented.

Risk factors for suicidal behaviour are:

- a history of psychiatric treatment
- a history of previous suicidal attempts
- alcohol dependency which is not controlled
- cocaine withdrawal
- a charge of homicide or a sexual offence
- youth.

For further details *section 3.6.*

Identifying depression

The features which are common in clinical depression are:

- an interrupted sleep pattern: usually patients wake in the early hours of the morning and are unable to get back to sleep
- lack of interest in daily living, and a general lethargy
- impairment of concentration
- low mood and a pessimistic view of life
- hopelessness about the future: this is a particularly worrying symptom as it usually precedes suicide
- increasing irritability
- poor appetite, although some people may nibble food throughout the day
- self-medication for depression or anxiety with drugs or alcohol which may then lead on to a dependency; it is important to assess whether depression pre-dated the alcohol or drug misuse.
- suicidal thoughts.

Identifying psychosis

Schizophrenia

Schizophrenia is the most common of the psychotic illnesses. It commonly begins to manifest itself in young adults, and as the prison population is comprised of predominantly young men, a prison doctor needs to bear in mind the possibility of an emerging psychosis if a prisoner presents as 'behaving oddly'. The young man may present as withdrawn and solitary, reluctant to communicate, or occasionally as aggressive and violent.

When interviewing a patient the doctor must aim for privacy with only a nurse present, and appear calm and unhurried and reassuring.

When making a mental state examination the following points need to be considered:

- **Behaviour:** does the patient conduct himself appropriately at interview? Staff may have reported unusual behaviour, for example prisoners laughing inappropriately, or spending long periods immobile on their beds, or apparently talking to someone who is not actually present.
- **Speech:** is it within normal expectations? Speech may be vague and difficult to follow, have apparent philosophical connotations, and indeed sometimes be incomprehensible. This may be due to disturbances of thinking, such as thought blocking, or interpolations in the train of thought.

- **Mood:** the patient may appear depressed or anxious or irritable. Typically there is blunting of affect, or feelings, and sometimes, incongruity of affect, where the mood is not in keeping with the situation.

- **Hallucinations:** these are usually auditory, heard by the patients in their heads, and are very frequent in schizophrenia. The patient may describe one or more voices. The voices may be said to be giving a running commentary on what the patient is doing, or instructing him about what to do. Instructive voices may lead to a person killing himself or, more rarely, another person. It is therefore important to spend time and patience getting the history.

- **Delusions:** delusions are sometimes described as fixed beliefs, not in keeping with the normal and accepted beliefs in society. Persecutory delusions are common, and the patient may also experience delusions of reference or control. For example, the patient believes that rays are coming from a TV set and working in his brain to control some specific action. Fixed beliefs about one person may spread to include others, until a whole persecutory system is built up.

- **Attention and concentration:** this is usually affected by the other symptoms described, particularly the hallucinations. The patient finds it difficult to concentrate if the hallucinatory voices are also speaking to him, and this may be picked up during the interview.

Chronic schizophrenia

Schizophrenia usually continues to result in a general deterioration of the personality over time. The schizophrenic patient is often inactive, lacking drive, socially withdrawn, and emotionally apathetic, but modern medications and ongoing therapy are maintaining patients to a higher level of activity than in days gone by.

Identifying antisocial personality disorder (ICD-10: F 60.2)

Given the high prevalence of antisocial personality disorder among prisoners, prison doctors need to be aware of the condition, how it may present, and how it may be managed. The diagnosis of personality disorder can only be made with any degree of certainty if the symptoms have been present for two years or more. Personality disorder presents in late adolescence and is often preceded by childhood behavioural problems.

The common features of the antisocial personality disordered are:

- callous unconcern for the feelings of others
- persistent irresponsibility and disregard for social norms, rules and obligations
- failure to maintain enduring relationships, though having no difficulty in establishing them
- low tolerance to frustration
- low threshold for discharge of aggression and violence
- marked proneness to blame others.

It should be borne in mind that those affected may range from the relatively minor to the severely disordered. Those who are severely disordered may not be amenable to, or indeed express any wish for help. However, those of a lesser order, particularly if they are able to show some insight into the behaviour patterns which lead them into difficulties, can be helped in certain circumstances. Such treatment is best within a therapeutic community setting. The personality disordered can be highly manipulative, and firm boundaries need to be imposed. Staff working within a therapeutic community setting need to consult together frequently to avoid divisions; the patients are highly manipulative and delight in causing trouble between staff members, whilst they themselves remain smiling and untroubled!

Doctors and nurses must not lose sight of the fact that the personality disordered may become clinically depressed and require treatment for that; or they may have a dependency on alcohol or drugs and so require treatment for addiction. Indeed, a high percentage of those who become dependent on drugs have been found to have a personality disorder.

Managing mental illness in the prison context

Expert psychiatric advice and help are needed in all prisons, but most especially in all situations where prisoners are on remand or on trial. In some countries prisoners remanded into custody by the courts are held for many months in police custody, usually due to lack of prison spaces. These prisoners, in addition to those held in prison custody, also need regular access to a psychiatrist.

Evidence shows that the mentally ill are at a higher risk of being apprehended by the police than the rest of the community, and therefore their mental state needs to be confirmed and treated as soon as possible.

Prisons are not psychiatric hospitals, and any attempt to treat acutely mentally ill people in prison should be resisted. No patient should ever be treated in custody against his will unless it is to save his life (*section 2.6*). Any patient who is actively psychotic, and suffering from delusions and hallucinations, should be admitted to a community psychiatric hospital, at least until medication is established and he is in a quiescent stage of the illness.

Psychiatrists may argue that well-controlled or chronic patients are managed normally in the community, and that for a prisoner the prison is his community setting and he should be returned. A problem then arises because these chronic patients often cannot be safely managed in a normal prison location. Such patients may need to spend their time in a prison hospital or a special vulnerable prisoner unit. If that is the case, and chronic mentally patients are held in prisons, then arrangements must be made for them to have access to therapeutic outlets such as occupational therapy, art therapy, group work in skills training, and the like. They should not be locked in their cells for most of their day.

The prison doctor and the courts

The primary role of the prison doctor is the care of the prisoner/patient. He has no role to play in giving an opinion to a court about the mental state of his patient, or his risk of offending, or his dangerousness. The only possible exception to this advice is if the doctor believes it would be in the best interest of the patient for the court to have a psychiatric assessment. With the consent of the patient, he might then ask the court to arrange for this to be undertaken by an independent psychiatrist. Medical reports to the court should only be submitted by independent practitioners, ie. those not involved in treating the patients concerned (*section 2.19*).

Psychiatric side-effects of medications

Certain drugs prescribed for physical illnesses may have psychiatric side-effects. Some are well known:

- cardiovascular agents used to control hypertension
- some antibiotics, particularly if prescribed on an ongoing basis
- immunomodulators: including non-steroidal anti-inflammatory drugs such as salicylates, and corticosteroids (particularly if withdrawn too rapidly).

Others may not be well known as they have been introduced quite recently. These include:

- antiretroviral agents used for the treatment of HIV
- antiparkinsonian agents: up to 50% of patients with Parkinson's disease develop psychotic hallucinations, and up to 90% have symptoms of depression at some time
- epilepsy: one third of patients have psychosis or depression for varying periods directly related to the seizures, in addition to side-effects of medication itself.

3.5 Deliberate self-harm

Self-harm is a phenomenon observed primarily in young male and female prisoners. It usually takes the form of cutting to the anterior aspect of the wrists and forearms, although deliberate self-poisoning may occur. It is often repetitive; 20% repeating the act within 12 months.

Self-harming behaviour is indicative of a very distressed individual who is feeling unable to resolve his inner conflicts, and who is unable to communicate his feelings to others. Not only is the self-harming action an alternative means of communication, but it often seems to relieve some inner tension. The patient will often say that he 'feels better' after having cut himself.

Deliberate self-harm is usually a symptom of either family problems or family, interpersonal or intrapersonal problems. Some have a history of sexual abuse about which they have never spoken. Some are subjected to chronic bullying. Most self-harmers have a degree of clinical depression, although this may be masked.

Assessment

A thorough assessment, by a psychiatrist or an experienced psychiatric nurse, should always take place of any prisoner who self-harms. In prisons, the staff frequently tend to dismiss the incident as attention seeking (the question must be asked 'About what and why is he seeking attention?') and the patient may even be placed into unfurnished conditions that are indicative to him of punishment rather than care. This should never happen; it merely confirms to the patient his low self-esteem and worthlessness.

An assessment should include the following:

- The degree of suicidal intent; often the action has not been planned, but is a response to an ongoing saga of painful experiences.
- The possible explanation of the behaviour; this involves trying to discover the motivation for the self-harming act, and requires patience and time, possibly a long period of time, which is not always practicable.
- The problems experienced with family and peers.
- The presence of a psychiatric illness. The degree of depression must be determined, and also the degree of personality disorder. The co-existence of personality disorders with other mental disorders is common in the prison population, and those with borderline personality disorders are particularly prone to self-harm (section 3.4).
- The risks of further deliberate self-harm and of completed suicide. This involves a careful history and mental health assessment. A percentage of self-harmers go on to completed suicide. The high risk groups are the same as for suicide and are described in section 3.6.

Management

Ideally every prison should have available a multidisciplinary psychiatric team to draw up a management plan for these needy patients. This is rarely the case. The prison doctor and his healthcare team can, however, play an important part in reducing the patient's distress and helping him to see ways of resolving some of his conflicts.

The following should be part of a management plan:

- supervision
- intervening in a sympathetic way in a crisis
- increasing understanding of difficulties
- building a therapeutic relationship
- treating any coexisting disorders.

3.6 Suicide in prison

Suicide rates in the prisons of Western countries have increased relentlessly over the past 20 years. The rates are about four times higher than those in the general population, which have also increased. The suicide of a prisoner is one of the most distressing things that can happen. It is upsetting for the staff, particularly those who discover the body; it is upsetting for other prisoners; and it is upsetting for the relatives. All of these people experience guilt, believing that someone should have anticipated it, and should have done something to prevent it.

Identifying those who may be suicidal is, therefore, a big responsibility, and one which must be shared by all prison staff. Prison healthcare staff do not have the same contact with prisoners as the prison officers and other staff, who are working among the prisoners in the living units and in the work shops. It is these staff who will observe changes in behaviour or mood, and who have a responsibility to take appropriate action.

Suicide analyses

In any *general population*, for more than 90% of people who commit suicide one of the following will apply:

- affective disorder (50% of these are clinically depressed)
- schizophrenia
- alcohol or drug dependency
- 50–60% communicate suicidal intent in the week prior to suicide
- 80% see a physician within one month of dying.

The predictors of suicide in *affective disorders* are:

- hopelessness
- depressive turmoil, such as agitation, panic and delusional depression
- alcohol abuse
- suicidal ideation
- failed suicide attempts.

Links between *substance abuse* and suicide are increased by:

- comorbidity with depression or other psychiatric disorders
- poor medication compliance
- unsupported withdrawal from drugs or alcohol
- personal and/or psychosocial losses.

Of the prisoners who commit suicide, approximately:

- 33% have a previous psychiatric history
- 25% have had a previous inpatient psychiatric admission

- 33% have a history of alcohol abuse
- 20% have a history of drug abuse
- 50% have a history of self-harm.

The highest risk period for suicide to occur in prison is in the early days of incarceration. Remand prisoners are at particular risk. Half of suicides in prison occur in the first three months.

Prisoners vulnerable to suicidal behaviour

This group includes:

- those charged with homicide (10–20% of suicidal patients have a history of violence to others)
- those charged with sexual offences
- those facing long sentences
- the mentally ill
- the alcohol dependent.

Reception health screening

Given the above information, the importance of the reception health screening process cannot be over-emphasised (*section 2.4*). All receptions into custody should be interviewed at least by a nurse on the day of arrival, and by the prison doctor within 24 hours. In particular, it must be elicited if the prisoner has a history of:

- self-harm
- psychiatric treatment
- alcohol or drug misuse.

If there is a history of self-harm or psychiatric treatment in the past, it is advisable for the prison doctor to obtain a psychiatric opinion. Until this is happens, the prison doctor must decide whether the prisoner requires close supervision by healthcare staff, or whether he may be placed on a living unit and supervised by prison staff. The doctor will need to undertake a careful mental state examination, and in particular discover any suicidal ideation. If this is found to be the case, then the patient must be closely supervised. It is not advisable to locate a suicidal patient in a cell which has been stripped of all furnishings. He may not have an opportunity to commit suicide under these conditions, but the chances of doing so once the restrictions are eased are increased, and any trust between the healthcare staff and the patient is spoiled.

Some prisons train other prisoners to act as friends (listeners) and share a cell with someone who is thought to be at risk. This system seems to work well, and gets over the problem of not having staff available to sit with the 'at risk' cases. But there is no doubt that a highly suicidal prisoner should not be in prison but removed to a psychiatric hospital. Most prison hospitals are not equipped or staffed for the purpose, and are not suitable for nursing such patients.

Delay may be experienced in obtaining expert advice on the management of alcohol- and drug-dependent patients, and it is important that the prison doctor has knowledge on how to manage such cases in the first instance. Details of such assessment and treatment are to be found in *section 3.4.*

Training of staff

Prison doctors have a responsibility to ensure that prison

staff receive training about suicide awareness. Even within the vulnerable groups prisoners do not feel suicidal at all times, prison staff need to be aware of the stress factors that may trigger suicidal feelings, in addition to the behavioural signs that may need to be noted and investigated. This applies to all prisoners, as depression may go undetected, particularly in the young who tend to mask it. All staff must be taught to befriend those who are experiencing problems. More junior staff must also feel able to express any concerns to their superiors and the prison healthcare staff, who in turn have a responsibility to investigate further.

Particular factors which may occur during imprisonment and trigger suicidal feelings

- **Isolation:** prison doctors should visit the isolation units of the prison on a regular basis.
- **Fear:** prisoners should be encouraged to verbalise any fears.
- **Loneliness:** this is common early in a custodial offence.
- **Breakdown of relationships:** prison staff should be alert to information about this.
- **Bullying:** prison healthcare staff should be alert to signs that a patient may have been bullied.
- **Inactivity:** every effort should be made to engage prisoners in work, education, physical exercise, etc. on a daily basis.
- **Loss of hope for the future:** intelligent listening may elicit evidence of this.

- **Guilt/shame:** this is common in homicide cases.
- **Not realising that help is available:** prison staff should always make it clear that they are available to talk to prisoners. A system whereby prisoners are designated to specific officers is helpful.

Particularly stressful occasions which occur in prison

Particularly stressful occasions are:

- entering prison for the first time
- unexpected bad news
- getting into debt
- an expected visit not materialising
- unexpected transfer to another prison
- sentencing, particularly if a long sentence is imposed.

Signs of stress or despair

Signs of stress and despair of the patient include:

- spending more time alone
- becoming withdrawn and uncommunicative
- not eating
- not sleeping
- not planning for the future (eg. for approaching home leave)
- bursts of anger over trivialities
- increasing visits to the healthcare centre for consultations with healthcare staff.

Preventive measures

It is important for each prison to have in place a policy and strategy for identifying and managing suicide. The policy should be based on Compassion, Cooperation, Care, and Communication. It should include the establishment of:

- A coordinating suicide committee, drawn from all grades of staff and chaired by a senior staff member.
- Staff training arrangements for all grades of staff who will have contact with prisoners, that includes:
  - an awareness of the factors listed above which increase prisoner stress
  - signs of stress to be further investigated
  - the importance of listening, and training in intelligent listening
  - asking about suicidal thoughts
  - the importance of sharing the concerns with other staff and the medical staff
  - following up each case and not assuming the responsibility lies with someone else
  - involving the prison population in the strategy, and training some prisoners to be listeners.
- A formalised system setting out the action to be taken by staff at every stage.
- Regular reviews.

Management of the suicidal patient

It is important for staff to know of their particular responsibilities in relation to all suicidal prisoners. In particular, every member of staff should know the suicide policy and should have received training in suicide awareness as described above. This training should be reinforced at regular intervals. All staff should be trained in the use of resuscitation equipment, which should be available and readily accessible to all staff, and each staff member should be aware of how to proceed if a suicide is discovered.

Categorisation of risk

It is useful to categorise the suicidal into three levels of risk.

Risk level 1:
The actively suicidal, requiring constant observation

These are patients who admit suicidal plans and who may have made serious attempts at self-harm. Such patients should be transferred to a psychiatric facility, but if this cannot be arranged they remain the responsibility of the prison healthcare staff. The patient should be kept under constant visual observation. This does not need to be in isolation from other patients providing a nurse is present at all times. Difficulties may arise during the night hours in the prison context when all prisoners are located in locked rooms. The prison doctor will need to negotiate with the governor of the prison, to devise a way in which this might be achieved. One way is to arrange for other trusted and trained prisoners to share a room with the suicidal patient, and to take turns at remaining awake and if necessary talking to the patient. The prisoners should be able to summon prison staff help at any time, but in any case a staff member should visit the cell at 15-minute intervals. If the patient will accept night sedation, this may help.

A review of each patient must take place at least every 24 hours, when his mental state is assessed and decisions taken as to who should be involved in his care. The advice of a psychiatrist must certainly be sought, and it is also useful to involve a clinical psychologist and an occupational therapist. A careful and thorough handover of information between staff at the time of shift changes should be ensured. Medication may be initiated, but within the prison context this cannot be administered against the will of the patient. If a patient does accept medication then strict observance must take place to ensure that he complies and swallows it, to avoid the possibility of it being stored towards a suicide attempt.

Risk level 2:
The recently suicidal, requiring 15-minute supportive observation

These are patients who are judged not to be actively suicidal, but who in the recent past have made suicidal attempts, who have expressed suicidal ideation, and who are still contending with losses or other stressor factors. A designated member of the healthcare staff should know of the whereabouts of these patients at all times, and the patients should be in the presence of either healthcare staff or inmates at all times. All staff should be made aware of any prisoner who is on 15-minute supportive observation. Daily support in the form of psychotherapy or cognitive therapy should be in place, and bi-weekly reviews should continue.

Risk level 3:
Those in a vulnerable prisoner group requiring support

These are patients identified as belonging to an increased risk category, but who are not judged to be currently suicidal. They may be resident on the living units, but all staff should be aware of their vulnerability, and keep a particularly watchful brief. They may need continuing therapeutic support on an outpatient basis.

3.7 Vulnerable prisoner groups

Definition

The *Concise Oxford Dictionary* definition of the word vulnerable as 'susceptible to injury'. In one sense all prisoners are vulnerable to the unique pressures encountered within the prison environment, the main one being loss of autonomy.

The role of the prison doctor

The prison doctor can help to alleviate the general vulnerability of all prisoners by the way in which he approaches them. There are certain principles that apply:

- A non-judgemental approach, treating all patients with respect, and listening attentively to what they say.
- Empowering patients by discussing diagnosis and treatment options.
- Having a good knowledge of the common disorders encountered in prison health care; and having a willingness to seek a second opinion.
- Making it clear that he is a personal physician, acting solely on behalf of the prisoner who is his patient.
- Making it clear to all that in the clinical setting confidentiality will be respected.
- Maintaining privacy for all consultations.

Factors which increase the vulnerability in prisoners

These include:

- **Reduced capacity to understand instructions and requirements:** such prisoners may have a degree of learning disability, which often goes undetected in prisoners; or they may be misusing drugs of addiction; or they may be psychotic; or they may be foreign nationals who are not familiar with the language. It is useful to provide a pamphlet for each prisoner on entry into a prison, that is written in simple plain language, and which details the services offered by the healthcare department. It should be available in a range of languages (*section 2.4*).

- **Disempowerment:** due to poor clinical practice within the prison setting which does not allow for privacy and confidentiality when clinical interviews are taking place.
- **Belonging to a minority group, either ethnic or cultural:** such groups may include sexual minorities such as homosexuals, ethnic minorities, and cultural minorities such as travellers.
- **Previous life experiences:** that may include torture and child abuse, resulting in excessive fear of the prison environment.

Some prisoners are particularly susceptible to mental or physical abuse, either from other prisoners; or from unthinking, uncaring or prejudiced prison staff; or indeed from the system itself. For example, many prison systems treat juveniles and young prisoners as adults, not taking into account their immaturity and the United Nations Convention on the Rights of the Child (1990) (see *Annex 1*). Women prisoners also face discrimination; they are a minority group (80% of prisoners are men) and the policies and strategies of most prison administrations are male orientated. The mentally ill are also at particular risk in the normal prison setting, as are those with learning difficulties. (All prisons provide separate units for the young and for women, but the conditions on these units are often inferior to those provided for the adult men, and in his role as adviser on health matters, the prison doctor should do all he can to bring pressure to bear with the governor to improve such situations.

This chapter does not deal with these groups specifically but it concentrates on prisoners who are likely to be subjected to abuse from fellow prisoners, and who are removed from normal locations, either to special vulnerable prisoner accommodation or to seclusion units, such as punishment units, for their protection.

These include prisoners who are:

* charged with offences of physical and mental child abuse
* charged with any sexual offence, especially paedophilia
* bullied on account of their inadequacy in some area, either physical, mental, or emotional
* in debt to other prisoners eg. on account of drug dealing
* homosexuals, transsexuals or transvestites, who may be used for the sexual gratification of other prisoners.

Prison doctors should take an interest in prisoners who are so held in protection, not only on the grounds of humanity, but also to monitor their mental state. They should also be alert, from their consultations with prisoners, to the possibility of abuse. Abused prisoners may readily sink into a depression and become suicidal. But this is also an area where the doctor is not only a personal clinician to an individual patient, but is also an advocate on behalf of these groups of prisoner. Prison doctors should urge the prison authorities to provide specific and adequate accommodation that enables removal of these prisoners from the threat of harm, and provides routines that meet their needs, in general, providing work and relaxation therapy; and should specifically provide sex offender programmes for paedophiles. The prison doctor should make a point of visiting all segregation units of the prison on a regular basis, and make sure he is available to any prisoner who wishes to consult with him.

Transsexual prisoners

A transsexual person is convinced that he or she is of the gender opposite to that indicated by their external genitalia, and has an overpowering wish to live as a member of that opposite sex. Transsexualism is rare but it is encountered in prisons.

The immediate problem that presents is one of location, because as a general rule the transsexual prisoner is located in an institution appropriate to his birth gender. Moreover, transsexual people are usually persistent in their demands for medication to change their sexual characteristics, and so they come to the attention of prison doctors early on in their custody. First and foremost the prison doctor should seek advice from an expert in the subject. As a general rule if gender-altering medication has been started prior to imprisonment then it should be continued, but if it has not then very careful thought should be given to commencing it while the person is in custody. If the prisoner wishes to proceeds with surgery this is even more problematic, so it should be delayed if at all possible. The transsexual prisoner must usually seek refuge in a vulnerable prisoner unit or in the prison healthcare centre if a bed is available. Doctors and nurses require immense patience to manage transsexual patients and need to acquaint themselves with the condition and in particular the compulsive nature of the desire to change sex.

Paedophile prisoners

Paedophiles are attracted not to adult sexual partners but to children, and this attraction does not change over time. 'Treatment' of paedophiles who have offended is directed towards teaching self-control and avoidance techniques. Group therapy, behaviour therapy, and aversion therapy are the usual tools. Prison doctors have only a limited role to play in these treatments, because they are usually carried out by psychologists.

Hormonal medication has been advocated from time to time, and has been used extensively at Herstedvester prison in Denmark, which deals exclusively with the treatment of sex offenders of all types. As a general rule, however, hormonal medication, that suppresses sexual drive, raises ethical concerns within the prison setting as it is difficult to be sure that the consent of the sexual offender is freely given and no element of coercion is present.

Given that the release of the prisoner from custody often hinges on the risk of re-offending, it may be argued that medication is only accepted by the prisoner to effect release, and will be discontinued by the prisoner as soon as he is released. If aggression plays a part in the offending behaviour, then reduction of the sex drive may still not be sufficient to deter offending.

Certainly long-term supervision of offending paedophiles after release from custody is required, and is necessary to reduce the risk of re-offending. This is the responsibility of community social workers and probation officers, and calls for close liaison and cooperation between the prison service and the external authorities well before these sex offenders are released.

Homosexual prisoners

The prison doctor or nurse has no specific part to play other than that of being a confidante and adviser. In western countries homosexuality is not illegal, but in countries where this is not the case Doctors and nurses must take care not to breach confidentiality. The doctor does, however, have a duty to exhort the prison governor to make condoms available to *all* prisoners – homosexual prisoners are likely to enter into sexual relations with other homosexuals, and prisoners who are not usually homosexual may become sexually active in the predominantly all-male environment of a prison (*section 3.2*). If possible abuse of an individual homosexual comes to the notice of the doctor, the doctor has a duty to inform the governor of his suspicions, without breaking patient confidentiality, and to insist that staff take action (*sections 2.16, 3.3*).

Drug-dependent prisoners

Most drug-dependent prisoners manage to get access to drugs, but the drugs have to be paid for by one means or another. This payment may be with money, in kind, or by services rendered, sometimes sexual ones. Drug-dependent prisoners who get into debt may require protection. It is crucial for the good order of any prison that access to drugs is limited, and a constant vigil is required to limit the drugs that enter the prison. It is equally important for treatment to be available to help dependent drug users either to become abstinent or to receive maintenance opiate medication. Those who are drug-free should be helped to remain so (*section 3.1*).

3.8 Hunger strike

Definition

This involves deliberate and persistent total or partial refusal of food by a mentally competent person with the intention of protesting to effect some change, either in regimens or privileges, or to obtain perceived rights.

The need for medical care of prisoners who persistently refuse food in order to make a protest is rare but challenging for the prison health care staff. Knowledge about the hunger strike quickly spreads and gets into the political arena. Governments want to resist the demands, which often have political overtones, but also do not want prisoners to die because of fear of the backlash of public opinion, and the consequences. Pressure is therefore brought to bear on the doctor to keep the prisoners alive, if necessary, by force feeding.

The most important guidance for prison doctors regarding hunger strikes is the Declaration on Hunger Strikers that was adopted by the 43rd World Medical Assembly in Malta in November 1991, and editorially revised at the 44th World Medical Assembly in Marbella, Spain in September 1992.

To summarise the declaration: a doctor must obtain consent from the patient before applying any skills to assist him. The only exception is in an emergency when the patient is incapable of giving consent. Because the end stage of food refusal is coma, it follows that the patient is not then capable of giving consent, and it is possible to argue that the doctor may then intervene by artificial feeding, to save the patient's life. However, this is not the case if the patient has made it clear that he refuses intervention to prevent death. Any doctor who cannot accept this ultimate non-intervention should make it clear at an early stage to the patient; the patient is then entitled to be attended by another physician.

Management of food-refusing patients

Every inmate who is refusing food should be interviewed by the doctor, and the cause for the refusal ascertained. Mental illnesses, such as psychosis, depression, and anorexia nervosa all need to be excluded. It is always wise to get a second opinion from an independent psychiatrist as to soundness of mind, in every case of food refusal. Indeed it is helpful if the prison doctor is in contact with independent professional colleagues such as a psychiatrist and specialist physician, for support and advice throughout the hunger strike, providing it is he, the prison doctor, who has the final responsibility.

If the doctor is satisfied that the patient is of sound mind, and has clarified the reason behind the hunger strike, then he has a duty to set out in detail to the patient, verbally and in writing, the consequences of pursuing the proposed course of action. The patient should be asked to sign a statement to the effect that he understands the consequences of his actions, and that he refuses all interventions. It should also be made clear to the patient that he is free to change his mind at any time.

The doctor must also decide the best location for the patient. Very soon after food refusal commences the patient should be persuaded to move to the prison healthcare centre or the prison hospital. In some cases a shared room can be helpful. Other prisoners are sometimes able to influence a food refuser to eat. However, single accommodation is usually preferable, particularly there is thought to be an element of coercion from other prisoners to maintain the fast. The most difficult hunger strikers to manage are those who are politically motivated. Dedication to their cause may be fanatical, but the degree of coercion may be great, as may the fear of possible repercussions from party leaders if the fast is not continued.

The prison doctor should visit the patient daily and should be alone. He should make clear that his conversations with the patient are confidential and that he fully respects the patient's decisions even if he wishes, as a carer, that it were otherwise. The patient is then far more likely to trust the doctor who at the very least can bring comfort and support.

If the patient agrees, regular follow-up examinations should take place, and these should cover:

- body weight
- body mass index (BMI, ie. weight in kilograms divided by the square of the height in metres)
- ketosis
- serum creatinine, electrolytes, uric acid, and blood count.

Each day the patient should be offered food and encouraged to drink 2–3 litres of fluid a day. It may be possible, if the patient agrees, to include electrolytes (containing 1.5 grams sodium chloride and 100 mmol potassium) and vitamin supplements. Consideration needs to be given to any pre-existing disorders such as diabetes mellitus, gout, gastritis, peptic ulcer, and any chronic disease. After discussing with the patient the complications of these conditions coexisting with starvation, decisions regarding treatment have to be made. It is important to point out to the patient that with the resulting onset of the severe central nervous system which takes place from the sixth week onwards in total fasting, no more decision-making will be possible. It is important to point out to the prisoner that because of the onset of severe central nervous system disorders (occur from the sixth week in total fasting) no more decision making will be possible. Any expression of will concerning life-saving medical measures must therefore be given and documented in good time.

As soon as weight loss of more than 10% of the initial body weight and a decrease of the BMI to below 16.5 is reached, permanent medical monitoring in a hospital unit will need to be enforced. If this is in another prison then a copy of the medical file of the patient, and any documented expression of the patient's instructions concerning life-saving medical measures after he has lost the capacity to decide or express his will, must be handed over to the medical team of the hospital.

The clinical course of fasting

Total refusal of fluids and food

Total refusal of fluids and food is extremely rare. Death will occur in a matter of days.

Total fasting with the ingestion of water only

As no calories, no vitamins, and virtually no electrolytes and trace elements are ingested, the body relies on its energy reserves, its deposits of fat and glycogen. The rapidly developing ketosis (a result of the accelerated beta-oxidation of fatty acids) suppresses the initial hunger pangs after the third day.

As the sensation of thirst is also reduced, insufficient fluid intake reduces the intake of sodium and as a result there is a reduction of extracellular fluid volume, resulting in circulatory problems. The glycogen reserves of the body are used up, and after about two weeks gluconeogenesis from amino acids sets in with the breakdown of essential tissues. This, together with the deficiency of thiamine, finally result in life-threatening cardiac arrhythmias and cardiac arrest as well as severe central nervous system disorders (ie. Wernicke's encephalopathy).

Without treatment or nutritional supplements, loss of competence for decision making and accountability is to be expected from the sixth week, and death is likely from the seventh week onwards. Survival has never been reported beyond the seventy-fifth day from the start of persistent total fasting.

The course of symptoms of total fasting (with ingestion of water only) are:

- **Day 1–3:** epigastric cramps and hunger pangs, which disappear after the third day.
- **Day 15 onwards:** aesthenia, fatigue, dizziness, feeling cold, euphoria and reduction or loss of the sensation of thirst.
- **Day 30 onwards:** bradycardia, hypotension, orthostatic hypotension, progressive oculomotor palsy, diplopia, strabismus and nystagmus, with excruciating nausea and vomiting. Nystagmus, and nausea and vomiting disappear as soon as the oculomotor palsy is complete, usually after one week
- **Day 40 onwards:** somnolence, cognitive impairment with loss of concentration and memory, mental confusion, stupor. At this point, competence for decision making and accountability ceases.
- **Subsequently:** haemorrhage of various tissues and organs, loss of hearing, Cheyne–Stokes respiration, extreme bradycardia and cardiac arrest.

Non-total fasting

Non-total fasting is abstention from solid food, but not from nutrition in liquid form such as milk, honey, dissolved sugar and vitamins. Non-total fasting may be practised by hunger strikers quite intentionally in order to prolong the period of the desired moral pressure. Its seriousness should not be underestimated because if continued for long enough it also can lead to the fatal disorders described above.

3.9 Death in prison custody

The doctor should seek to arrange for a terminally ill prisoner to die in the community rather than in prison. It is the last act of mercy that can be shown to a prisoner, and it is in keeping with maintaining human dignity.

Sudden deaths in custody should be certified by the prison doctor, and the cell should then be left undisturbed and locked. The prison authorities and the police should be immediately informed. They then assume responsibility for the body and for informing the patient's relatives of the death. The prison doctor should, however, offer his condolences to the family if he thinks fit. Any death that occurs in custody should be subject to a judicial autopsy and a public inquest.

3.10 Medical research in prison

Following the inhumane crimes committed against prisoners in the past, the majority of European states have effected laws that exclude prisoners from medical research. However, the AIDS epidemic and the rapid improvements in therapy as a result of clinical research have shown that the exclusion of prisoners from clinical phase III studies might put them at a disadvantage. Therefore exclusion is unethical.

Thus, subject to national legislation, it is recommended that prisoners should have access to clinical phase III studies, on condition that they are expected to produce a direct and significant benefit to the health of the prisoners, that no privileges are promised, that consent is free and independently obtained, and that all ethical principles concerning research on humans are strictly applied, particularly in relation to fully informed consent and confidentiality. All research studies carried out in prison must be subject to approval by an independent ethical committee or an alternative procedure guaranteeing these principles.

Research on the prevention, treatment and management of transmissible diseases in prison populations should be encouraged, provided that such research yields information which is not available from studies in the community. In all this research the same high ethical standards are to be observed and supervised by an independent outside ethical committees.

Annex 1

Annex 2

Annex 3

Annex One - International declarations, conventions and recommendations

Europe

Ethical and Organisational Aspects of Health Care in Prison. Recommendation No. R (98) 7. Adopted by the Committee of Ministers on 8 April 1998. Council of Europe, Strasbourg 1999

European Convention for the Prevention on Torture and Inhuman or Degrading Treatment or Punishment. Adopted by the Committee of Ministers on 26 November 1987 and entered into force 1 February 1989, Council of Europe, Strasbourg. (www.cpt.coe.int/en/docsref.htm)

European Convention on Human Rights. Council of Europe, Strasbourg 1952, 1963, 1966 (www.hri.org./docs/ECHR50.html)

European Prison Rules. Revised European Version of the Standard Minimum Rules for the Treatment of Prisoners. Recommendation No. R (87) 3. Adopted by the Committee of Ministers on 12 February 1987. Council of Europe, Strasbourg 1987. http://www.uncjin.org/Laws/prisrul.htm (accessed January 2006)

Medical Research on Human Beings. Recommendation No. R (90) 3. Adopted by the Committee of Ministers on 18 October 1993. Council of Europe, Strasbourg 1991

Prison and Criminological Aspects of the Control of Transmissible Diseases including AIDS and Related Health Problems in Prison. Recommendation No. R (93) 6. Council of Europe, Strasbourg 1995

Prison overcrowding and prison population inflation. Recommendation No. R (99) 22. Adopted by the Committee of Ministers on 30 September 1999. Council of Europe, Strasbourg 2001

United Nations

Basic Principles for the Treatment of Prisoners. Adopted by the General Assembly on 14 December 1990. United Nations, New York, 1991

Body of Principles for the Protection of Persons Under Any Form of Detention or Imprisonment. Adopted by the General Assembly on 9 December 1988. United Nations, New York, 1989. http://www.unhchr.ch/html/menu3/b/h-comp36.htm

Convention against Torture and Other Cruel, Inhuman or Degrading Treatment or Punishment. Adopted by the General Assembly on 10 December 1984 http://www.unhchr.ch/html/menu3/b/h_cat39.htm (accessed January 2006)

Convention on the Rights of the Child. Adopted by the General Assembly on 20 November 1989 (not yet ratified by all member states) http://www.unhchr.ch/html/menu2/6/crc/treaties/crc.htm (accessed January 2006)

International Covenant on Civil and Political Rights. Adopted by the General Assembly on 16 December 1966 and entered into force on 23 March 1976 http://www.unhchr.ch/html/menu3/b/a_ccpr.htm (accessed January 2006)

International Covenant on Economic, Social and Cultural Rights. Adopted by the General Assembly on 16 December 1966 and entered into force on 3 January 1976. United Nations, New York. http://www.ohchr.org/english/countries/ratification/3.htm (accessed May 2006)

Principles of Medical Ethics relevant to the Role of Health Personnel, particularly Physicians for the Protection of Detained Persons and Detainees Against Torture and Other Cruel, Inhuman or Degrading Treatment or Punishment. Adopted by the General Assembly on 18 December 1982. In: *Human Rights: A Compilation of International Instruments*. United Nations, New York, 1988. http://www.unhchr.ch/html/menu3/b/h_comp40.htm (accessed January 2006)

Prisons and AIDS: UNAIDS Point of View (UNAIDS Best Practice Collection). UNAIDS, Geneva

Standard Minimum Rules for Treatment of Prisoners. Adopted 1955, endorsed 31 July 1957 and effective implementation approved on 13 May 1977. In: *Human Rights: A Compilation of International Instruments*. United Nations, New York, 1987 http://www.unhchr.ch/html/menu3/b/h_comp34.htm (accessed January 2006)

The United Nations Rules for the Protection of Juveniles Deprived of their Liberty. Adopted by the General Assembly on 14 December 1990. United Nations, New York. http://www.ohchr.org/english/law/res45_113.htm (accessed May 2006)

The Universal Declaration of Human Rights. Adopted by the General Assembly on 10 December 1948. http://www.unhchr.ch/udhr/index.htm (accessed January 2006)

World Health Organization (WHO)

Guidelines for the Prevention of Tuberculosis in Healthcare Facilities in Resource-Limited Setting. WHO/TB/99.269. World Health Organization, Geneva 1999

Guidelines on HIV Infection and AIDS in Prison. World Health Organization: Geneva 1993

Prisons, Drugs and Society. A Consensus Statement on Principles, Policies and Practices WHO (Regional Office for Europe) Health in Prisons Project and the Pompidou Group of the Council of Europe: Berne 2001

Prison Health as Part of Public Health. Declaration of Moscow, 24 October 2003. WHO Regional Office for Europe: Geneva 2003

Status Paper on Prisons, Drugs and Harm Reduction. WHO Regional Office for Europe: Copenhagen 2005

World Medical Association (WMA)

Declaration Concerning Support for Medical Doctors Refusing to Participate in, or to Condone, the Use of Torture or Other Forms of Cruel, Inhuman or Degrading Treatment. Hamburg 1997. www.wma.net/e/policy/c19.htm (accessed January 2006)

Declaration of Edinburgh on Prison Conditions and the Spread of Tuberculosis and Other Communicable Diseases. Adopted by the World Medical Assembly, Edinburgh 2000. http://www.wma.net/e/policy/p28.htm (accessed January 2006)

Declaration of Helsinki. Recommendations Guiding Physicians in Biomedical Research Involving Human Subjects. Adopted June 1964, amended Tokyo 1975, Venice 1983,

Hong Kong 1989. Adopted by the World Medical Assembly, Fernay-Voltaire 1990 www.wma.net/e/policy/b3.htm (accessed January 2006)

Declaration of Tokyo. Guidelines for Medical Physicians Concerning Torture and Other Cruel, Inhuman or Degrading Treatment or Punishment in Relation to Detention and Imprisonment. Adopted by the World Medical Assembly, Tokyo in October 1975 and editorially revised Divonee-les-Bains in May 2005. http://www.wma.net/e/policy/c18.htm (accessed January 2006)

Declaration on Hunger Strikers. Adopted by the World Medical Assembly, Malta November 1991 and revised Marbella, September 1992. http://www.wma.net/e/policy/h31.htm (accessed January 2006)

Declaration on Hunger Strikers. Adopted by the World Medical Assembly, Edinburgh 1992. http://www.wma.net/e/policy/t1.htm (accessed January 2006)

Degrading Treatment. Adopted by the World Medical Assembly, Hamburg November 1997. http://www.wma.net/e/policy/c19.htm (accessed January 2006)

Oath of Athens. International Council of Prison Medical Services. Adopted by the World Medical Assembly, Athens 1979

Resolution on the Responsibility of Physicians in the Denunciation of Acts of Torture or Cruel or Inhuman or Degrading Treatment Of Which They Are Aware. Adopted by the World Medical Assembly, Helsinki 2003. http://www.wma.net/e/policy/t1.htm (accessed May 2006)

Statement on Body Searches of Prisoners. Adopted by the World Medical Assembly, Budapest October 1993 and editorially revised Divonee-les-Bains May 2005]. http://www.wma.net/e/policy/b5.htm (accessed January 2006)

The Istanbul Protocol. The Manual on Effective Investigation and Documentation of Torture and other Cruel, Inhuman or Degrading Treatment or Punishment. Adopted by the World Medical Assembly, Istanbul 1999. http://www.phrusa.org/research/istanbul_protocol (accessed January 2006)

Annex Two - Useful Websites

American Correctional Health Services Association at http://www.corrections.com/achsa

Centers for Disease Control and Prevention at http://www.cdc.gov

Council of Europe at http://www.coe.int

European Committee for the Prevention of Torture and Inhuman or Degrading Treatment or Punishment at http://www.cpt.coe.int

International Committee of the Red Cross at http://www.icrc.org

National Commission on Correctional Health Care at http://www.ncchc.org

Penal Reform International at http://www.penalreform.org

Physicians for Human Rightsat http://www.phrusa.org

Prison Health Care Practitioners at http://www.prisonhealthcarepractitioners.com

World Health Organization Regional Office for Europe at http://www.euro.who.int

World Health Organization Health in Prisons Project at http://www.hipp-europe.org

World Medical Association at http://www.wma.net

World Medical Association/Norwegian Medical Association at Web-based course
'Doctors working in prison: Human rights and ethical dilemmas' at http://lupin-nma.net

World Psychiatric Association at http://www.wpanet.org

International Centre for Prison Studies at http//www.prisostudies,org

Annex Three - Further Reading

Allen SA, Spaulding AC, Osel AM et al (2003) Treatment of chronic hepatitis C in a
state correctional facility. *Ann Intern Med* **138:**187–90

Backmund M, Meyer K, von Zielonka M, Eichenlaub D (2001) Treatment of hepatitis C
infection in injection drug users. *Hepatology* **34:**188–93

Bollini P (ed) (2001) *HIV in Prisons. A Reader with Particular Relevance to the Newly
Independent States.* World Health Organization, Regional Office for Europe, Geneva

Bone A (2000) *TB Control in Prisons – A Manual for Programme Managers.
WHO/TB/CDS/281.* World Health Organization, Geneva

Brockman B (1999) Food refusal in prisoners, a communication or a method of self-
killing? The role of the psychiatrist and resulting ethical challenges. *J Med Ethics*
25:451–56

Centres for Disease Control and Prevention (1996) Prevention and control of tuberculosis in correctional facilities. Recommendations of the advisory council for the
elimination of tuberculosis. *MMWR* 45(R8)

Davies DM, Ferner RF, de Glanville H (eds) (1997) *Davies Textbook of Adverse Drug
Reactions,* 5th edn. Oxford University Press, Oxford

Diazde S (ed) (2003) *Needle-Exchange in Prison.* Framework Program. Subdireccion
Direccion General de Instituciones Penitenciarias, Direccion General de Salud
Publica, Madrid

Faintuch J, Soriano FG, Ladeira JP et al (2000) Changes in body fluid and energy com-
partments during prolonged hunger strike. *Rev Hosp Clin Fac Med Sao Paulo*
55:47–54

Fazel F, Danesh J (2002) Serious mental disorder in 23 000 prisoners: a systematic
review of 62 surveys. *Lancet* **359:** 545–50

Fiellin DA, O'Connor PG (2002) Office-based treatment of opioid-dependent patients.
N Engl J Med **347:**817–23

Gordon H (2002) Suicide in secure psychiatric facilities. *J Adv Psychiatr Treat* **8:**408–17

Granich R, Binkin N, Jarvis W et al (1999) *Guidelines for the Prevention of Tuberculosis in
Healthcare Facilities in Resource-Limited Setting., WHO/TB/99.269.* World Health
Organization, Geneva

Hawton K, Catalan J (1987) *Attempted Suicide: A Practical Guide to its Nature and
Management,* 2nd edn. Oxford University Press, Oxford

ICD-10 Classification of Mental and Behavioural Disorders. World Health Organization,
Geneva 1992

International Corrections and Prisons Association (2001) *International Compendium of
Current Practices to Address Infectious Diseases in Prisons.* International Centre for
Criminal Law Reform and Criminal Justice Policy, Vancouver and The International
Corrections and Prisons Association, Ottawa

Kalk WJ, Felix M, Snoey ER, Veriawa Y (1981) Voluntary total fasting in political prisoners – clinical and biochemical observations. *S Afr Med J* **83**:391–94

Kosten TR, O'Connor PG (2003) Management of drug and alcohol withdrawal. *N Engl J Med* **348**:1786–95

Liebling A, Ward T (1994) *Deaths in Custody: International Perspectives*. Whiting & Birch, London

Lines R, Jurgens R, Stover H, Laticevschi D, Nelles J (2002) *Prison Needle Exchange: Lessons From a Comprehensive Review of International Evidence and Experience*. Canadian HIV/AIDS Legal Network. http://www.aidslaw.ca/Maincontent/issues/prisons.htm

Maher D, Grzemska M, Coninx R, Reyes H (1998) *Guidelines for the Control of Tuberculosis in Prisons. WHO/TB/98.250*. World Health Organization, Geneva 19

Morgan G, Owen J (1990) *Persons at Risk of Suicide*. Boots Company, Nottingham

Muscat R (2000) *Drug Use in Prison*. Council of Europe Publishing, Strasbourg

Paterson A (1930) Paterson on prisons. In: Ruck SK (ed) (1951) *The Collective Papers of Sir Alexander Paterson*. Frederick Muller, London

Paton J, Jenkins R (eds) (2002) *Mental Health Primary Care in Prison*. Royal Society of Medicine Press, London

Peel M (1997) Hunger strikes: Understanding the underlying physiology will help doctors provide proper advice. *Br Med J* **315**:829–30

Penal Reform International (2001) *Making Standards Work. An International Handbook on Good Prison Practice*, 2nd edn. Penal Reform International, The Hague (French translation published by Penal Reform International, Paris 1997)

Reyes H, Coninx R (1997) Pitfalls of tuberculosis programmes in prisons. *Brit Med J* **315**:1447–50

Royal College of Psychiatrists (2002) *Vulnerable Patients, Vulnerable Doctors*. Royal College of Psychiatrists, London

Stern V (ed) (1999) *Sentenced to Die? The Problem of TB in Prisons in Eastern Europe and Central Asia*. International Centre for Prison Studies, King's College, London